Evaluation of Potential Employee Exposures at a Medical Examiner's Office

Bradley S. King, MPH, CIH
Elena Page, MD, MPH

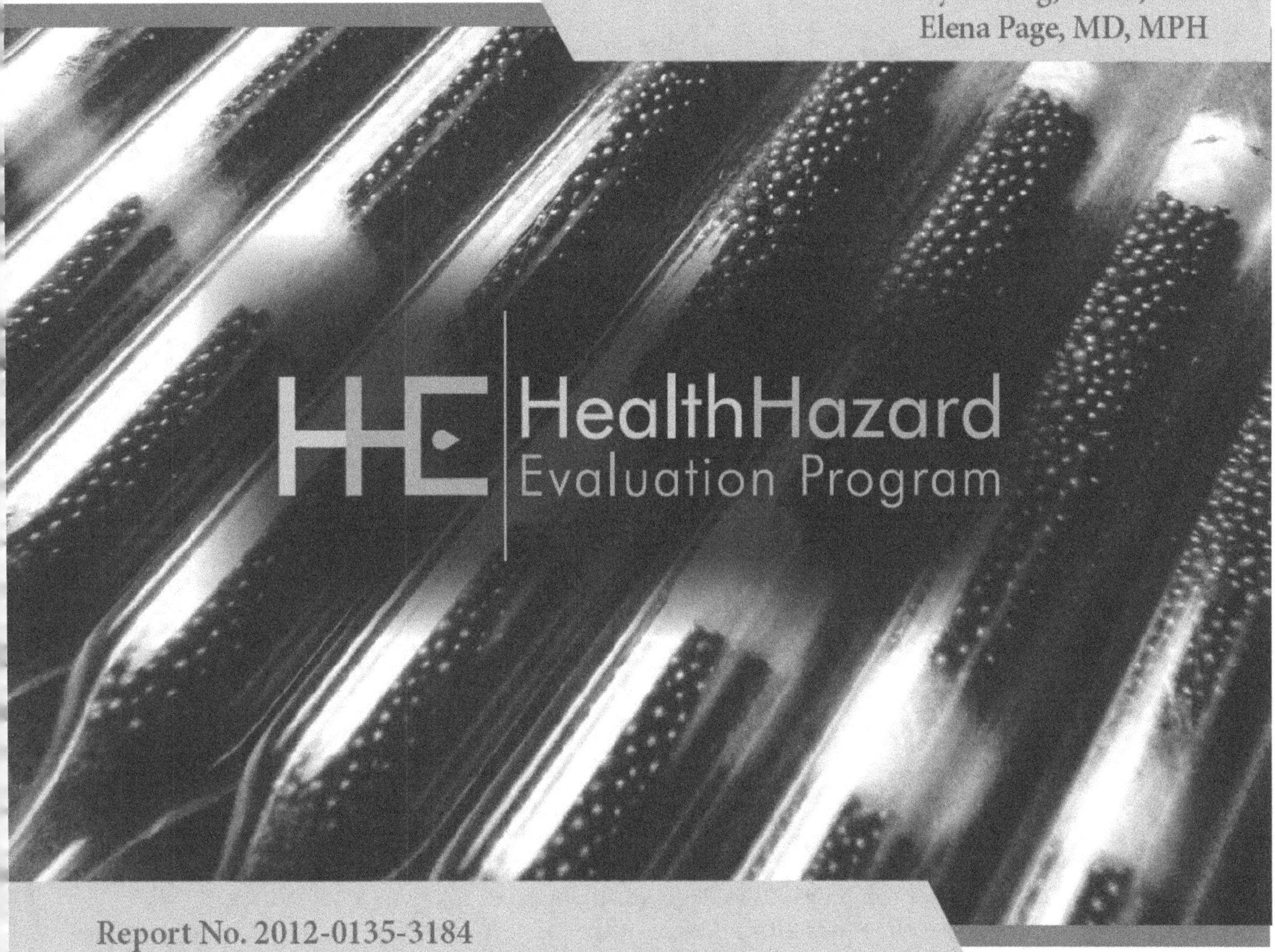

HHE | HealthHazard
Evaluation Program

Report No. 2012-0135-3184
June 2013

U.S. Department of Health and Human Services
Centers for Disease Control and Prevention
National Institute for Occupational Safety and Health

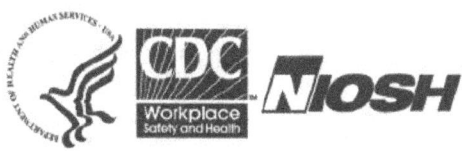

Contents

The cover photo is a close-up image of sorbent tubes, which are used by the HHE Program to measure airborne exposures. This photo is an artistic representation that may not be related to this Health Hazard Evaluation.

Highlights of this Evaluation

The Health Hazard Evaluation Program received a request from employer representatives at a medical examiner's office. The request was submitted because of concerns that employee health problems such as hives, acquired angioedema, itchy eyes, mouth sores, asthma, and gastrointestinal symptoms, among others, may have been related to the environmental conditions at the facility.

What We Did

- We evaluated the facility in May 2012.

- We interviewed employees about their work and health.

- We observed work practices and procedures in the autopsy suite, histology laboratory, and toxicology laboratory.

- We sampled the air for formaldehyde and particles during five autopsies.

- We sampled the air for formaldehyde and volatile organic compounds during tissue prepping and processing in the histology laboratory and for volatile organic compounds in the toxicology laboratory.

- We collected surface samples for mold throughout the building, including inside the ventilation system.

- We collected surface samples for fiberglass throughout the building.

- We measured temperature and relative humidity in several areas.

> We evaluated exposures to volatile organic compounds, mold, airborne particles, and formaldehyde in the autopsy suite, histology laboratory, and toxicology laboratory of a medical examiner's office. Exposures to formaldehyde and volatile organic compounds were below occupational exposure limits. However, poor indoor environmental quality conditions (e.g., mold growth, water incursion) were present and may be related to respiratory problems reported by employees. Recommendations were made to address the causes of the poor indoor environmental quality conditions.

What We Found

- Some employees reported respiratory problems that may be related to exposures in the workplace.

- Other health problems such as kidney stones, acne, hives, and bladder infections were not related to the building.

- Temperatures and relative humidity varied by building area and some levels fell outside of recommended ranges.

- Employees used powdered latex gloves. Airborne latex particles could contribute to allergic symptoms.

- Formaldehyde exposures in the autopsy suite were below occupational exposure limits.

- Air change rates in the autopsy suite exceeded national guidelines. Air flowed into the autopsy suite from the adjacent room as recommended.

What We Found (continued)

- Exposures to volatile organic compounds in the histology and toxicology laboratories were very low.

- Chronic water damage was found throughout the building.

- Mold growth and deteriorating duct lining were found in the ductwork that served floors 1–3.

- Disintegrated fiberglass was found in surface samples but few intact fiberglass fibers were present.

What the Employer Can Do

- Purchase local exhaust ventilation units for cranial autopsy saws.

- Identify and repair all leaks from the building's pipes, windows, roof, and façade.

- Maintain consistent and comfortable temperatures and airflow throughout the building.

- Remove mold safely from the ductwork to prevent spreading mold spores through the building's ventilation system.

- Provide nitrile gloves instead of powdered latex gloves.

- Evaluate the potential for entrainment of morgue exhaust into rooftop air intakes.

- Tell employees about steps being taken to address indoor environmental quality problems.

What Employees Can Do

- Use local exhaust ventilation during cranial autopsies when available.

- Stop using powdered latex gloves. Use nitrile gloves instead.

- Keep containers of formaldehyde closed except when needed during autopsies.

- Report any health and safety concerns to your supervisor and to your doctor.

- Become active in the health and safety committee. Attend meetings and take any training related to your job.

Mention of any company or product does not constitute endorsement by NIOSH. In addition, citations to websites external to NIOSH do not constitute NIOSH endorsement of the sponsoring organizations or their programs or products. Furthermore, NIOSH is not responsible for the content of these websites. All web addresses referenced in this document were accessible as of the publication date of this report.

Abbreviations

°F	Degrees Fahrenheit
ACGIH®	American Conference of Governmental Industrial Hygienists
ANSI	American National Standards Institute
ASHRAE	American Society of Heating, Refrigerating, and Air-Conditioning Engineers
C	Ceiling limit
CFR	Code of Federal Regulations
EPA	Environmental Protection Agency
HHE	Health hazard evaluation
HVAC	Heating, ventilating, and air-conditioning
IEQ	Indoor environmental quality
MDC	Minimum detectable concentration
MQC	Minimum quantifiable concentration
NIOSH	National Institute for Occupational Safety and Health
OEL	Occupational exposure limit
OSHA	Occupational Safety and Health Administration
PEL	Permissible exposure limit
ppm	Parts per million
REL	Recommended exposure limit
sp.	Species
STEL	Short-term exposure limit
TWA	Time-weighted average
VOC	Volatile organic compound
WHO	World Health Organization

Introduction

The Health Hazard Evaluation Program received a request from a manager at a medical examiner's office. The request concerned possible health hazards associated with work practices and workplace conditions in several areas including the autopsy suite, the toxicology and histology laboratories, and offices. Specific exposures of concern included volatile organic compounds (VOCs), fiberglass, mold, particulates, and formalin (a preservative containing formaldehyde). Concerns of poor indoor environmental quality (IEQ) and insufficient ventilation were also reported. We evaluated the building in May 2012.

Facility Description

The medical examiner's office provided a variety of forensic services for death investigations involving criminal violence, suicide, or accidents as well as deaths that occurred in a correctional facility or in a suspicious or unusual manner. The headquarters building where these services were performed opened in 1960. It had six floors above ground, and a basement and cellar below ground; it included an autopsy suite, mortuary, toxicology and histology laboratories, and offices. The medical examiner's office also occupied a second facility nearby; many of the employees working there had previously worked at the headquarters building.

The autopsy suite was located in the basement. Several rooms in the cellar below the basement were used to store files, stock jars holding tissue and formalin, and other items. The autopsy suite was supplied with 100% outdoor air filtered through a prefilter and a high efficiency particulate air filter that was ducted from an intake off the second floor. From the second floor heating, ventilating, and air-conditioning (HVAC) unit, air moved through ductwork to supply storage rooms in the cellar, including the stock jar storage room. These areas in the cellar acted as plenums before the air was transferred to the basement-level autopsy suite and other areas by transfer fans. Within the autopsy suite were eight downdraft autopsy tables and a ducted lab hood that provided additional exhaust for the autopsy suite. Additionally, three air recirculating units were used in the autopsy suite to supplement the main ventilation system. Exhaust from the basement-level autopsy suite and morgue was ducted to exhaust vents on the roof.

Offices took up most of the first, second, and third floors. The original HVAC design used two fans on the second floor to provide supply air to these three floors. One fan had been decommissioned, leaving the other fan to supply the three floors with a mixture of fresh and recirculated air. The facility's engineers were unable to provide information about the amount of outdoor air being provided by the operating fan or why the second fan was decommissioned. Return air from these floors mixed with fresh air, passed through the fan and heating/cooling coils in the air handling unit, and was divided into separate "hot deck" or "cold deck" ductwork. The ductwork directed the air into mixing boxes in individual offices on the three floors. Some of these mixing boxes had thermostats controlling a plunger that determined the amount of hot or cold air entering the room. However, not all thermostats in offices were functioning, and the parts to fix them reportedly were difficult to find or no longer available.

Personnel in the fourth floor histology laboratory worked with tissues collected during autopsies, processing them for microscopic examination of the tissue cells. Personnel in the toxicology laboratory on the fifth and sixth floors evaluated drugs, poisons, and other toxic compounds in body fluids and tissues. Floors four, five, and six were supplied with 100% outdoor air by two supply fans on the roof; the air was ducted directly to ceiling vents on each floor. The air supplied to the rooms on these floors was then exhausted directly outside. The supply air was heated by a hot water system that used reheat coils. Electric thermostats controlled these coils by regulating hot water supplied to the reheat coils. An actuator in the thermostat opened a valve; it was reported that the valves and the actuators were failing. New valves had been located to replace those that were malfunctioning or had failed. Replacement actuators reportedly were unavailable.

In addition to the main ventilation systems, several rooms on multiple floors had independent perimeter air supply units. Each perimeter unit had a heating and cooling coil and a self-contained fan unit that pulled air from the space between the inner and outer façade walls of the building into the room. Pleated paper filters were present in some units. Some of these filters reportedly had not been replaced in years. Following past renovation work, access to the internal equipment for several of the perimeter units was obstructed.

Work Process Descriptions

The autopsy suite had the capacity for eight simultaneous autopsies, each performed by a medical examiner with medical residents and mortuary technicians assisting as needed. Activities during autopsies could expose the autopsy team to chemical and biological hazards. For example, when the autopsy team opened the chest cavity to remove and examine the internal organs, organ tissue samples were removed and placed in open containers of a 10% neutral buffered formalin solution. This solution was used to fix and preserve tissue specimens for histologic examination. To access brain tissue, the skull cap was removed with a hand-held oscillating autopsy saw. No local exhaust ventilation was used. Four or five autopsies typically were performed per day, with ten autopsies performed on a busy day. Approximately 30 employees worked in the autopsy suite.

Investigations of drugs and poisons in body fluids and tissues occurred in the toxicology laboratory on the fifth and sixth floors. Laboratorians used techniques such as gas chromatography/mass spectrometry to analyze blood, urine, body tissues, stomach contents, and other specimens for chemicals. Twenty employees worked in this laboratory.

The histology laboratory received tissue specimens collected during autopsies. The tissues, maintained in small cassettes, were removed from the formalin solution held in the containers and loaded into a tray for further processing. This work typically was done within a chemical fume hood. Further processing removed the tissue fluids and replaced them with alcohol and paraffin to fix the tissue in a block of paraffin. Chemicals used in the tissue processing included dehydrants such as ethyl, isopropyl, and methyl alcohol, and aliphatic hydrocarbons. After processing, the block was sliced and the tissue slices were mounted on a slide, dyed, and viewed under a microscope. Twelve employees worked in this area.

Methods

Interviews

The director of employee health and safety provided a roster of all 160 employees at the headquarters building and a list of seven employees who worked at the second facility nearby and had reported medical issues they felt were related to work at the headquarters building. We serially selected every third employee from the headquarters building roster for confidential in-person medical interviews. All employees at the headquarters building received an e-mail to notify them that we would be available if they wished to be interviewed but had not been selected. We also interviewed employees from the second facility and one retired employee by phone or in person. We asked about work location, job duties, health issues they felt were related to work, medical history, smoking history, and potential stressors at work. In addition, a complete medical history was taken to determine if any medical issues employees had but did not relate to their work could be unrecognized occupational illnesses. Medical records were obtained and reviewed for employees who reported work-related health issues for which they had received medical evaluation.

Autopsy Suite Exposures

On May 22, 2012, we observed work practices and procedures during five autopsies in the basement autopsy suite. We sampled the air for formaldehyde on eight employees over a full shift according to the National Institute for Occupational Safety and Health (NIOSH) Method 2016, with modifications [NIOSH 2010]. A medical examiner and a medical resident also wore a second sampler to collect 15-minute breathing zone air samples. A 15-minute area air sample was also collected between the first and second round of autopsies near one of the autopsy tables to document background concentrations of formaldehyde. For the 15-minute formaldehyde samples, the minimum detectable concentration (MDC) was 0.008 ppm (parts per million) and the minimum quantifiable concentration (MQC) was 0.025 ppm for an air volume of 3 liters. For the full shift formaldehyde samples, the MDC was 0.001 ppm and the MQC was 0.004 ppm for an air volume of 19.5 liters.

Because the oscillating saw creates airborne particulate matter, two Hach Ultra Analytics Met One HHPC-6 Handheld Airborne Particle Counters were placed near autopsy tables to measure the concentration of airborne particles. We measured air velocity with a TSI Q-Trak™ model 9565-P Indoor Air Quality Meter and probe model 966 for calculation of the number of air changes per hour. We used Nextteq smoke tubes to visualize air flow patterns and assess pressure differentials. We used a TSI Q-Trak™ model 9565-P Indoor Air Quality Meter with probe model 982 for environmental temperature and relative humidity measurements.

Toxicology Laboratory Exposures

On May 23, 2012, we assessed exposures in the toxicology laboratories. We observed employees doing blood extractions, preparing working solutions, handling buffers and other chemicals, screening urine, and working on the gas chromatography/mass spectrometry instruments. We collected air samples on thermal desorption tubes to screen for VOCs according to NIOSH Method 2549 [NIOSH 2010]. We collected full-shift air samples on three employees and area air samples for analysis of specific VOCs according to NIOSH Method 1501 [NIOSH 2010]. Environmental temperature and relative humidity measurements were made using Q-Trak™ models 7565-X and 9565-P Indoor Air Quality Meters with probe model 982.

Histology Laboratory Exposures

On May 23 and 24, 2012, we assessed exposures in the histology laboratory. We observed a laboratory associate preparing autopsy tissues and took full-shift air samples for formaldehyde and VOCs. Additionally, we collected seven 15-minute, short-term breathing zone air samples for formaldehyde on the lab associate. During the 2 days of sampling she spent most of her time removing tissue cassettes from formalin-holding jars and placing them in a metal tray for processing. We also observed other laboratory employees sectioning paraffin blocks. Three full-shift air samples for VOCs were collected, one each on a laboratory helper, a microbiologist, and the laboratory director. Area air samples were taken for VOCs around the laboratory. Two full-shift air samples for formaldehyde were also collected on the laboratory helper and microbiologist. Sampling and analysis of formaldehyde was done according to NIOSH Method 2016, with modifications; sampling and analysis for VOCs was done according to NIOSH Methods 2549 and 1501 [NIOSH 2010]. Environmental temperature and relative humidity measurements were made using a Q-Trak™ model 7565-X Indoor Air Quality Meter.

Indoor Environmental Quality

On May 24, 2012, we collected 10 surface samples for mold from locations throughout the building, including the second floor HVAC unit and on ductwork, window ledges, carpet, and walls of second, third, fourth, and sixth floor rooms. We collected six samples for fiberglass from surfaces such as desks and window sills in rooms 125, 311, 333, and 613 and in hallways on the third and sixth floors. Stick-to-it clear plastic microscope slides were used to collect the surface mold and fiberglass samples. Immediately prior to use, the slide was removed from the slide mailer, and its protective liner was peeled off to expose the adhesive. The slide was placed adhesive side down, gently pressing down to ensure contact was made between the slide and the surface. The slide was then removed from the surface, with the adhesive side of the slide pulling mold spore structures, hyphae, and fiberglass from the sampled surface. The slides were packed in individual mailers, shipped to the analytical laboratory, and analyzed microscopically.

We collected temperature and relative humidity measurements on the first, third, and sixth floors with Q-Trak™ models 7565-X and 9565-P Indoor Air Quality Meters to determine if these parameters fell within established guidelines.

Results

Interviews

We interviewed 53 employees. Of these, 40 were serially selected from the roster (none refused to be interviewed), six asked for interviews, six were from the second facility, and one was retired. Of the 53, 33 reported they had no health issues they related to their work at the headquarters building. One reported sarcoidosis, but did not feel it was related to work. Twenty employees reported health concerns they related to work at the headquarters building. The most common symptoms were eye irritation (five); nose irritation, congestion, and sneezing (six); exacerbation of allergies (four); and sinus problems (three). Four individuals reported having been diagnosed with asthma since beginning work at the headquarters building. Other symptoms reported were headache, cough, hives and angioedema (two each); and wheeze, skin problems, stress due to odors from the morgue, dental problems, leg and arm cramps, acne, and kidney stones (one each). Medical records were reviewed for five employees. One record showed a diagnosis of occupational asthma due to mold exposure. The other records did not show sufficient evidence to document a work-related condition.

Autopsy Suite Exposures

During the five autopsies observed, air samples were taken for formaldehyde on three medical examiners, two medical residents, and three mortuary technicians. Results of these samples are presented in Appendix A, Table A1. No short-term concentrations of formaldehyde exceeded applicable ceiling or short-term occupational exposure limits (OELs) set by the Occupational Safety and Health Administration (OSHA), NIOSH, or the American Conference of Governmental Industrial Hygienists (ACGIH). Full-shift, time-weighted average (TWA) concentrations ranged from 0.01–0.03 ppm and were well below the OSHA permissible exposure limit (PEL) of 0.75 ppm. Some full-shift TWA concentrations were above the NIOSH recommended exposure limit (REL) of 0.016 ppm.

Aerosol measurements were taken using direct-reading instruments mounted at the feet of autopsy tables 4 and 7. Results are shown in Figures B1 and B2 in Appendix B. Background aerosol concentrations (measured in particles/liter of air) are shown beginning at 9:14 a.m., before autopsy procedures started. Most background particles measured were in the size range of 0.3–0.5 micrometers in diameter. A source of additional aerosols produced during the autopsies was using the oscillating saw to cut through the cranial bone to remove the skull cap. No local exhaust ventilation was used during this procedure. Aerosol concentrations showed small peaks when the oscillating saw was used. Typically, bone cutting with the saw lasted no longer than 5 minutes. While small peaks were observed when the saws were in use, aerosol levels returned to background levels fairly rapidly after the saws stopped.

Ventilation measurements were taken at the eight downdraft tables and one fume hood. On the basis of these exhaust measurements and the measured dimensions of the room, the calculated air changes per hour for the room was 20. This is above the minimum recommended of 12 air changes per hour for autopsy rooms [Facility Guidelines Institute 2010; ASHRAE 2011]. Smoke tube testing identified a negative pressure differential between the autopsy room and the adjacent rooms as recommended to minimize the spread of contamination.

During autopsies, we observed employees using face shields, nitrile or latex gloves, aprons, scrubs, booties, and head covers. N95 filtering facepiece respirators, appropriate for autopsy procedures, were used correctly and in accordance with the OSHA respiratory protection standard.

Toxicology Laboratory Exposures

We collected two area air samples to screen for VOCs. Compounds identified near two gas chromatography/mass spectrometry instruments included ethyl benzene and xylene isomers, toluene, and heptane. Compounds identified in the extraction room included ethyl benzene and xylene isomers, toluene, heptane, butyl chloride, and ethyl acetate. On the basis of these screening samples, ethyl benzene, xylenes, toluene, ethyl acetate, benzene, and heptane were quantified from three full-shift air samples and one area air sample. All concentrations measured were at or below 0.14 ppm, the highest concentration, which was for ethyl acetate. The breathing zone concentrations of VOCs were below 1/100 of the most conservative OEL. Laboratory personnel wore nitrile gloves, a laboratory coat, and safety glasses.

Histology Laboratory Exposures

We collected one full-shift and seven 15-minute short-term air samples for formaldehyde on a laboratory associate while she prepared, processed, and fixed tissue samples. We also collected two full-shift air samples, one each on a laboratory helper and a microbiologist. Results of these samples are presented in Appendix A, Table A2. No short-term personal breathing zone air sample results for formaldehyde exceeded ceiling or short-term OELs set by OSHA, NIOSH, or ACGIH. Results of full-shift TWA concentrations were well below the OSHA PEL; one of the full-shift TWA concentrations was slightly above the NIOSH REL.

VOCs were used in the tissue processor. Screening air samples showed low levels of ethyl benzene and xylene isomers, toluene, ethyl acetate, and isopropanol. Other compounds identified included ethanol, benzene, and heptane. On the basis of these screening samples, ethyl benzene and xylene isomers, toluene, ethyl acetate, benzene, and heptane were quantified from three full-shift air samples and one area air sample. All concentrations measured were at or below 0.11 ppm, the highest concentration recorded for one of the compounds (xylenes). The breathing zone concentrations of every compound for which we sampled were below 1/100 of the most conservative OEL.

Employees preparing, processing, and fixing tissue samples wore nitrile inner gloves and powder-free latex outer gloves, a laboratory coat, and an apron. Employees slicing paraffin blocks and mounting the slices on slides wore gloves and a laboratory coat.

Indoor Environmental Quality

Ten surface samples were collected at locations on the second, third, fourth, and sixth floors for the presence of mold growth. The ductwork immediately beyond the second-floor HVAC unit that serves the building's first three floors appeared to have a large amount of deteriorating material contaminated with mold (Appendix B, Figure B3). Other locations sampled included those where water incursions had been reported. Results of the microscopic analysis of the tape samples are detailed in Appendix A, Table A3. Concentrations of fungal structures are semi-quantitative (i.e., rare, few, moderate, and many). Identification was facilitated by the observation of spores, hyphae, and conidia. Predominant fungi identified included *Alternaria* species (sp.), *Aureobasidium/Hormonema* sp., *Aspergillus/Penicillium* sp., *Cladosporium* sp., *Engyodontium/Tritirachium* sp., *Myxomycete/Periconia*-like sp., *Penicillium* sp., *Scytalidum*-like sp., and *Ustilago/Ustilaginoid* sp.

Examinations of the slides from six surface samples from rooms on the first, third, and sixth floors showed trace amounts of intact fiberglass on each sample. However, each sample contained material that appeared to be rough-edged glass slag, perhaps a result of fiberglass breakage. Cellulose fibers were also prominent along with various plant fibers and pieces.

We measured temperature and relative humidity in several areas. Results are shown in Appendix A, Table A4. The indoor temperatures ranged from 65 degrees Fahrenheit (°F) in the autopsy suite to 78°F in the toxicology laboratory. The recommended temperatures ranges are 68°F–75°F for autopsy rooms and 70°F–75°F for laboratories (including general and histology laboratories) [ANSI/ASHRAE/ASHE 2008]. The relative humidity ranged from 53% in an office on the third floor to 71% in an office on the sixth floor, above the 65% level recommended by the American National Standards Institute/American Society of Heating, Refrigerating, and Air-Conditioning Engineers (ANSI/ASHRAE) [ANSI/ASHRAE 2010a].

We also observed the following problems at the headquarters building:
- Possible short circuiting of air because supply diffusers and exhaust grilles were close to one another
- Long runs of ductwork to a single supply diffuser at the end of the ductwork resulting in low airflow
- Locations in the building with multiple supply diffusers but few exhaust grilles
- Inability to access certain perimeter air supply units for maintenance and repairs

We received reports of inconsistent airflow throughout the building and the inability of the HVAC system to remove heat produced by the laboratory equipment, particularly on the fifth and sixth floors. The buildings' engineers reported difficulty in locating parts to replace old, malfunctioning HVAC system components. Additionally, employees reported the presence of body decomposition odors on the upper floors of the building. Air intakes for these floors and the morgue exhaust were on the roof making it possible for exhaust air to be entrained into the outdoor air intakes.

Discussion

We identified several occupational health and safety-related problems in the headquarters building including use of powdered latex gloves, chronic water intrusion or excessive moisture throughout the building, inadequate housekeeping, and the poor condition of the HVAC system. Some employees reported work-related health problems shown to be associated with occupancy in damp or moldy buildings, including upper and lower respiratory symptoms and asthma. Respiratory irritation, allergies, asthma, and nasal congestion could be related to airborne latex particles from the use of powdered latex gloves, microbial contamination from chronic water damage, ventilation problems related to issues in the system's design and control, inadequate housekeeping and building maintenance, or temperature and relative humidity levels outside of established IEQ guidelines. Some evidence in the medical literature shows that sarcoidosis may be related to damp or moldy buildings [Newman et al. 2004; Rossman et al. 2008; Newman and Newman 2012]. Some health problems reported by employees are not related to exposure in the building, such as kidney stones, acne, and bladder infections.

Cornstarch is used to powder sterile and non-sterile natural rubber latex gloves to aid in glove donning. Natural rubber latex proteins alone or glove powder containing such proteins can become airborne and represent a health hazard. Glove powder in environmental dusts also can pose a hazard. The three main types of reactions to latex-containing objects include irritant contact dermatitis, allergic contact dermatitis, and immediate hypersensitivity [NIOSH 1997a]. Additional information on the occupational hazards associated with these exposures can be found in the NIOSH Alert, "Preventing Allergic Reactions to Natural Rubber Latex in the Workplace" at http://www.cdc.gov/niosh/docs/97-135/ [NIOSH 1997a].

Allergic responses are the most common type of health problem associated with exposure to molds. These may include sneezing; itching of the nose, eyes, mouth, or throat; nasal stuffiness and runny nose; and red, itchy eyes. These were the most commons symptoms reported by employees. In 2009, the World Health Organization (WHO) published guidelines for protection of public health from mold and other exposures in damp buildings [WHO 2009]. On the basis of its review of the scientific literature for this report, WHO concluded that there was sufficient epidemiologic evidence that occupants of damp buildings are at risk of developing upper and lower respiratory tract symptoms (including cough, wheeze, and dyspnea), respiratory infections, asthma, and exacerbation of asthma. At least one employee had a documented diagnosis of occupational asthma due to mold in the workplace, and three others reported having been diagnosed with asthma since beginning work at the headquarters building. WHO also concluded that limited evidence suggests associations between bronchitis and allergic rhinitis and damp buildings. They noted clinical evidence that exposure to mold and other microbial agents in damp buildings is associated with hypersensitivity pneumonitis. Mold is not the only exposure that may be present in damp buildings, and it is still unclear exactly what exposures in damp buildings are responsible for health effects [WHO 2009]. In addition to mold, dust mites, bacteria, and chemical emissions can be present [NIOSH 2012].

No exposure guidelines for mold in air exist, so it is not possible to distinguish between "safe" and "unsafe" levels of exposure. Nevertheless, the potential for health problems is an important reason to prevent indoor mold growth and to remediate indoor mold contamination. Moisture intrusion, along with nutrient sources such as building materials or furnishings such as carpet and upholstered furniture, allows mold to grow indoors, so it is important to keep the building interior and furnishings dry. NIOSH concurs with U.S. Environmental Protection Agency (EPA) recommendations to remediate mold contamination in indoor environments found at http://www.epa.gov/mold/mold_remediation.html [EPA 2001; Redd 2002].

The location that had the most mold was the ductwork immediately after the second floor HVAC unit. All four samples collected in this location had a variety of mold species at levels described as "moderate" to "many." The ductwork provided a pathway for dissemination of mold spores to other locations in the building. Samples collected at other locations showed less mold contamination. Additional information on health effects and mold remediation can be found in the Centers for Disease Control and Prevention document "Mold Prevention Strategies and Possible Health Effects in the Aftermath of Hurricanes and Major Floods" at http://www.cdc.gov/mmwr/preview/mmwrhtml/rr5508a1.htm [Brandt et al. 2006].

One of the most common deficiencies in the indoor environment is the improper operation and maintenance of ventilation systems and other building components [Rosenstock 1996]. The combination of heat-producing equipment and poor HVAC performance can affect occupant comfort through increased environmental temperatures. In addition to reported water incursion directly into the building, high relative humidity can create a damp environment capable of supporting mold growth. Measured temperature and relative humidity fell outside recommended ranges for specific areas of the facility. Improved HVAC operation and maintenance, higher ventilation rates, and comfortable temperature and relative humidity can potentially improve occupant symptoms even when a specific cause-effect relationship is not identified.

Employees in the autopsy suite faced a number of potential occupational hazards inherent in their work, including exposures to infectious agents [CDC 2012]. All autopsies involve potential exposures to blood and other body fluids, a risk of being splashed or splattered upon, and a risk of percutaneous injury [Nolte et al. 2002]. Exposure to sharp objects within the body and bone fragments may also result in cuts, and the manipulation of large organs may result in body splashes [CDC 2012]. During these procedures, autopsy suite employees may be at risk of exposure to infectious agents such as *Mycobacterium tuberculosis* and bloodborne pathogens such as Hepatitis B and C, and human immunodeficiency virus [Nolte et al. 2002].

Procedures that involve the use of mechanical devices (e.g., oscillating saws) may create airborne particles that contain infectious pathogens such as *Mycobacterium tuberculosis* as well as those not normally transmitted by the inhalation route; such particles can also contaminate inanimate surfaces [Nolte et al. 2002]. Skull cap removal potentially generates high concentrations of infectious aerosols [Green and Yoshida 1990]. Droplets of blood and cerebrospinal fluid as well as the interstices of bone matrix may contain these infectious agents, but they could also be carried on the surface of particles formed by the combination of bone dust particles with fluid droplets [Green and Yoshida 1990]. The median diameter of bone dust particles in the breathing zone of a saw operator generated during a cranial autopsy has been reported to be 0.37 micrometers, which can easily penetrate the alveolar region of the lung and can remain airborne for long periods [Green and Yoshida 1990]. Our data show the majority of particles measured were in the size range of 0.3–0.5 micrometers in diameter and that peaks in aerosol concentrations were produced during use of the oscillating saw. No local exhaust ventilation was used in conjunction with the oscillating saw. NIOSH evaluations of cranial autopsies done with and without the aid of local exhaust ventilation indicate that using local exhaust ventilation significantly reduced exposure to aerosols produced by the saws [NIOSH 1997b].

Formaldehyde in formalin solution is the most common chemical to which autopsy employees are exposed [CDC 2012]. Common health complaints due to exposure to low concentrations of formaldehyde include irritation of the eyes, nose, and throat; nasal congestion; headaches; skin rash; and asthma [NRC 1981]. It often is difficult to attribute specific health effects to particular concentrations of formaldehyde because some people may have symptoms at levels where others may experience no symptoms [NRC 1981].

Formaldehyde concentrations during 15-minute short-term sampling periods in the autopsy suite and histology laboratory were below short-term or ceiling limits. All full-shift exposures were below the OSHA PEL; several results in the autopsy suite were slightly above the NIOSH REL. However, this REL was established in 1981 when NIOSH first recognized formaldehyde as a potential occupational carcinogen. On the basis of the carcinogen policy at the time, NIOSH set the REL to the "lowest feasible concentration," which for formaldehyde was defined as the analytical limit of quantification of 0.016 ppm for up to a 10-hour TWA and a ceiling limit of 0.10 ppm that should not be exceeded [NIOSH 1981]. Research has shown, however, that concentrations of formaldehyde in ambient air often can approach or exceed this level [Lemen 1987]. Additionally, a revision of the NIOSH carcinogen policy [NIOSH 1995], combined with better exposure characterization and advances in risk assessment and management strategies, support the need for NIOSH to reassess the formaldehyde REL. Nevertheless, the continued use of exposure controls in the autopsy suite, such as downdraft tables, and efforts to reduce the amount of time during which formaldehyde-containing jars are open are important in minimizing these exposures. The use of a chemical fume hood for tissue preparation appears to be useful in limiting the quantity of formaldehyde exposures.

Conclusions

Water incursion, mold growth, high relative humidity, HVAC system deficiencies, use of latex gloves, and poor maintenance and housekeeping practices may be contributing to some of the health problems reported by employees. These include respiratory irritation, allergies, asthma, and nasal congestion. Implementing the recommendations below will address such deficiencies and may reduce the quantity and severity of symptoms experienced by employees.

Recommendations

On the basis of our findings, we recommend the actions listed below. We encourage the medical examiner's office to use a labor-management health and safety committee or working group to discuss our recommendations and develop an action plan. Those involved in the work can best set priorities and assess the feasibility of our recommendations for the specific situation at the headquarters building of the medical examiner's office.

Our recommendations are based on an approach known as the hierarchy of controls (Appendix C: Occupational Exposure Limits and Health Effects). This approach groups actions by their likely effectiveness in reducing or removing hazards. In most cases, the preferred approach is to eliminate hazardous materials or processes and install engineering controls to reduce exposure or shield employees. Until such controls are in place, or if they are not effective or feasible, administrative measures and/or personal protective equipment may be needed.

Engineering Controls

Engineering controls reduce employees' exposures by removing the hazard from the process or by placing a barrier between the hazard and the employee. Engineering controls protect employees effectively without placing primary responsibility of implementation on the employee.

1. Provide local exhaust ventilation when using cranial autopsy saws during autopsies. Mobile bone dust collection systems that attach to a variety of cranial autopsy saws and provide high efficiency particulate air filtration are commercially available.

Administrative Controls

The term administrative controls refers to employer-dictated work practices and policies to reduce or prevent hazardous exposures. Their effectiveness depends on employer commitment and employee acceptance. Regular monitoring and reinforcement are necessary to ensure that policies and procedures are followed consistently.

1. Identify and repair all points of water incursion in the building, including leaks originating from the building's pipes, windows, roof, and façade.

2. Remove mold contamination in the ventilation ductwork in a manner that would prevent aerosolization and distribution of mold spores through the ventilation system.

3. Improve the operation and maintenance of the HVAC systems to provide appropriate ventilation rates and temperatures. This includes providing resources to replace or renovate aspects of the building's HVAC systems determined to be past their useful working life including failing or non-functioning thermostats and other temperature-setting equipment. The inability to find replacement parts for necessary components is a problem that needs to be addressed.

4. Ensure the temperature and relative humidity in the building follow current guidelines for office, autopsy suites, and laboratory spaces [ANSI/ASHRAE/ASHE 2008; ANSI/ASHRAE 2010a].

5. Evaluate the appropriateness of the ductwork design, including the locations of supply and exhaust registers, to ensure that proper supply and exhaust of conditioned air meets the needs of the specific areas of the building.

6. Improve housekeeping and maintenance practices. In particular, we observed stained and dirty carpet, upholstery, and air supply registers. Remove and replace soiled carpet if it cannot be adequately cleaned and provide more resources to maintain a greater level of housekeeping throughout the building.

7. Replace lids on containers of formalin as soon as possible after using.

8. Evaluate the potential that exhaust from the morgue is being entrained into air intakes on the roof. If necessary, take corrective action such as relocating exhaust or air supply vents.

9. Start an IEQ management program. An IEQ manager or administrator with clearly defined responsibilities, authority, and resources should be selected. This individual should have a good understanding of the buildings' structure and function, and should be able to communicate effectively with employees. Although no comprehensive regulatory standards specific to IEQ have been established, guidelines have been developed by organizations and agencies, including ASHRAE, NIOSH, and the U.S. EPA.

10. Include an employee representative in the IEQ management program to assist with communication. The NIOSH/U.S. EPA document, "Building Air Quality: A Guide for Building Owners and Facility Managers" may be helpful. A companion NIOSH/U.S. EPA guide, "Building Air Quality Action Plan," discusses how to develop and assess an IEQ management program.

11. Encourage employees with potential work-related health concerns to report their concerns to their supervisors and to seek evaluation and care from a healthcare provider who is knowledgeable in occupational medicine and IEQ issues.

12. Inform building occupants of the actions taken to address IEQ problems and the rationale for decisions made to address these problems.

Personal Protective Equipment

Personal protective equipment is the least effective means for controlling hazardous exposures. Proper use of personal protective equipment requires a comprehensive program and a high level of employee involvement and commitment. The right personal protective equipment must be chosen for each hazard. Supporting programs such as training, change-out schedules, and medical assessment may be needed. Personal protective equipment should not be the sole method for controlling hazardous exposures. Rather, personal protective equipment should be used until effective engineering and administrative controls are in place.

1. Use nitrile gloves for dermal protection during work activities in lieu of powdered latex gloves.

Appendix A: Tables

Table A1. Air sampling results for formaldehyde in the autopsy suite, May 22, 2012

Sample location	PBZ/Area	Sampling period (minutes)	Short-term TWA concentration (ppm)	Full-shift TWA concentration (ppm)
Medical examiner #1	PBZ	412	NA	0.02
Medical examiner #2	PBZ	402	NA	0.03
Medical examiner #3	PBZ	424	NA	0.02
	PBZ	15	[0.02]	NA
	PBZ	15	[0.01]	NA
	PBZ	15	0.04	NA
	PBZ	15	0.02	NA
	PBZ	15	ND	NA
Medical resident #1	PBZ	430	NA	0.03
Medical resident #2	PBZ	16	[0.01]	NA
	PBZ	15	0.03	NA
	PBZ	15	0.04	NA
	PBZ	15	[0.02]	NA
	PBZ	15	[0.02]	NA
	PBZ	15	[0.02]	NA
Mortuary technician #1	PBZ	413	NA	0.01
Mortuary technician #2	PBZ	400	NA	0.01
Mortuary technician #3	PBZ	246*	NA	0.02
Autopsy table	Area	16	ND	NA
NIOSH REL [NIOSH 2010]			C 0.1	0.016
OSHA PEL [NIOSH 2010]			STEL 2.0	0.75
ACGIH TLV [ACGIH 2012]			C 0.3	—

Values in brackets indicate levels between the MDC and the MQC.

C = Ceiling

NA = Not applicable

ND = Not detected

PBZ = Personal breathing zone

STEL = Short-term exposure limit

*Represents less time than a typical full-shift period due to the employee finishing the shift early

Table A2. Personal breathing zone air sampling results for formaldehyde in the histology laboratory, May 23–24, 2012

Sample location	Sampling period (minutes)	TWA concentration for 15-minute samples (ppm)	TWA concentration (ppm)
Laboratory helper	413	NA	0.01
Microbiologist	376	NA	0.02
Laboratory associate	351	NA	0.01
	16	ND	NA
	15	[0.01]	NA
	15	ND	NA
	15	0.04	NA
	15	0.06	NA
	15	0.03	NA
	15	0.03	NA
NIOSH REL [NIOSH 2010]		C 0.1	0.016
OSHA PEL [NIOSH 2010]		STEL 2.0	0.75
ACGIH TLV [ACGIH 2012]		C 0.3	—

Values in brackets indicate levels between the MDC and the MQC.

For the 15-minute samples, the MDC was 0.008 ppm, and the MQC was 0.025 ppm on the basis of an air volume of 3 liters.

For the full-shift samples, the MDC was 0.001 ppm, and the MQC was 0.004 ppm on the basis of an air volume of 19.5 liters.

C = Ceiling

NA = Not applicable

ND = Not detected

STEL = Short-term exposure limit

Table A3. Surface sampling results for mold, May 24, 2012

Sample location	Rare	Few	Moderate	Many
Ductwork after 2nd floor HVAC unit	Pollen		*Cladosporium*	*Aureobasidium/ Hormonema* *Engyodontium/ Tritirachium*
Ductwork after 2nd floor HVAC unit	—	—	*Scytalidum* Hyaline hyphae	*Cladosporium* *Alternaria* *Ustilago* Dematiaceous hyphae Dematiaceous conidia/ spores Hyaline conidia/spores
Ductwork after 2nd floor HVAC unit	—	—	—	Hyaline hyphae Hyaline conidia/spores
Ductwork after 2nd floor HVAC unit	—	Hyaline hyphae Hyaline conidia/spores	Dematiaceous hyphae	Dematiaceous conidia/spores
Room 218 ductwork in women's restroom	—	Hyaline hyphae Hyaline conidia/spores	Dematiaceous condia/spores	*Cladosporium*
Room 309 window ledge	*Epicoccum*	*Myxomycete/ Periconia* Dematiaceous conidia/spores Plant hairs	Pollen	—
Room 324 window ledge	*Pithomyces/ Ulocladium* *Epicoccum*	Ascospores *Cladosporium* Hyaline conidia/spores	Dematiaceous conidia/spores *Myxomycete/ Periconia* Pollen	—
Room 404 carpet on floor	—	—	—	Bacterial cocci
Room 405 near wall replacement	*Alternaria/ Pithomyces* *Polythrincium*	*Aspergillus/ Penicillium* Hyaline conidia/spores	—	—
6th floor toxicology lab wall baseboard	Hyaline conidia/ spores Dematiaceous conidia/ spores Pollen	*Aspergillus/ Penicillium* *Myxomycete/ Periconia* Algae	Yeast	—

Table A4. Temperature and relative humidity measurements, May 22–24, 2012

Sample location	Date	Sampling period	Temperature (°F) range and [average]	Relative humidity (%) range and [average]
Autopsy suite	05/22	8:30 a.m. – 2:26 p.m.	65–68 [67]	59–62 [59]
Room 335	05/22	8:35 a.m. – 4:03 p.m.	74–77 [75]	53–57 [55]
Anthropology room 324	05/22	8:40 a.m. – 4:10 p.m.	73–75 [74]	54–59 [57]
Histology laboratory room 415	05/23	8:15 a.m. – 12:59 p.m.	74–75 [75]	62–67 [65]
Toxicology laboratory near room 503	05/23	8:17 a.m. – 2:28 p.m.	76–76 [76]	59–62 [60]
Toxicology laboratory room 508	05/23	8:24 a.m. – 12:48 p.m.	77–78 [77]	57–60 [58]
Room 125	05/24	9:27 a.m. – 12:16 p.m.	73–75 [74]	54–59 [56]
Anthropology room 324	05/24	9:35 a.m. – 12:07 p.m.	69–69 [69]	63–67 [65]
Room 613	05/24	9:33 a.m. – 12:03 p.m.	70–71 [71]	68–71 [69]

Appendix B: Figures

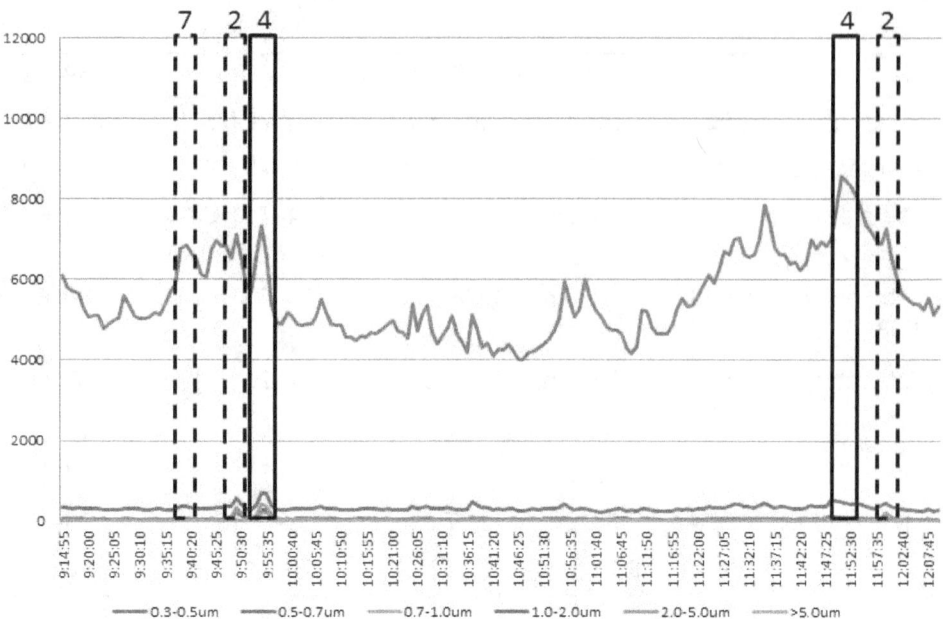

Figure B1. Concentration of aerosols at the foot of table 4 in the autopsy suite during five autopsies. Figure B1 shows two solid-line boxes, labeled 4, which represent the time when the oscillating saw was used at autopsy table 4 where the first particle counter was mounted at its foot. Figure B1 also shows three dashed-line boxes, labeled 7 or 2, which represent the times when an oscillating saw was used at other autopsy tables (table 7 for the first dashed-line box and table 2 for the second and third dashed-line boxes) in the autopsy suite.

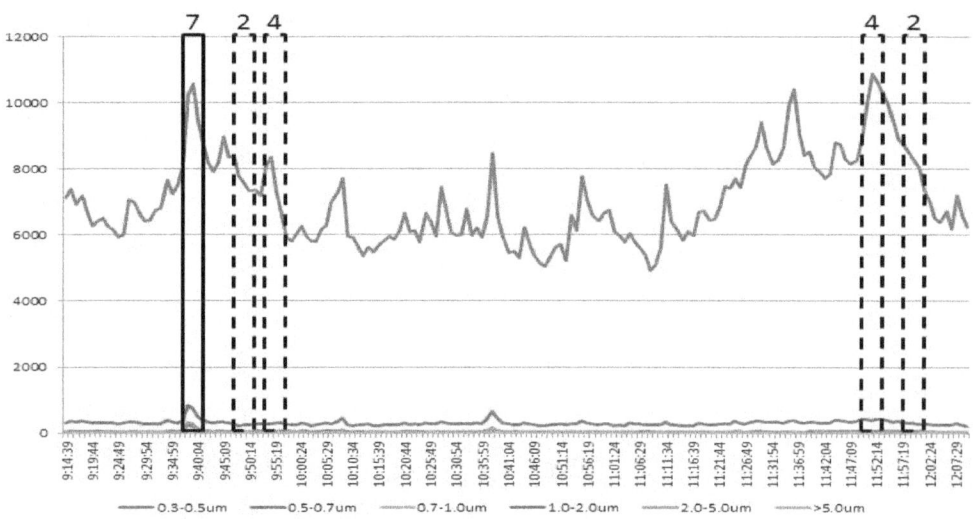

Figure B2. Concentration of aerosols at the foot of table 7 in the autopsy suite during five autopsies. Figure B2 shows one solid-line box, which represents the time when the saw was used at autopsy table 7 where the second particle counter was mounted at its foot. Figure B2 also shows four dashed-line boxes, labeled 2 or 4, which represent the times when the saw was used at other autopsy tables (table 2 for the first and fourth dashed-line boxes and table 4 for the second and third dashed-line boxes).

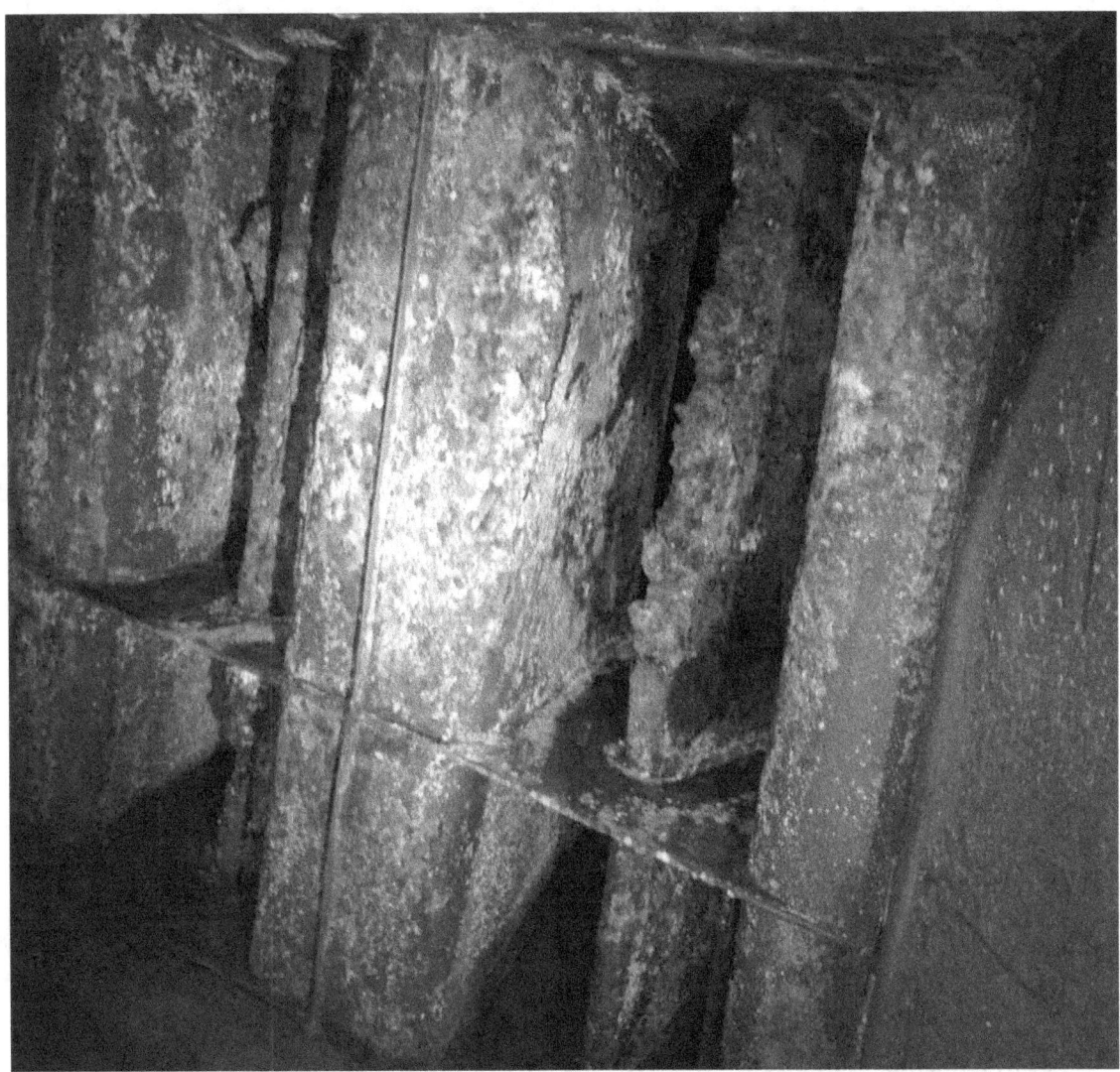

Figure B3. Deteriorating material and mold growth in the 2nd floor HVAC unit ductwork.

Appendix C: Occupational Exposure Limits and Health Effects

NIOSH investigators refer to mandatory (legally enforceable) and recommended OELs for chemical, physical, and biological agents when evaluating workplace hazards. OELs have been developed by federal agencies and safety and health organizations to prevent adverse health effects from workplace exposures. Generally, OELs suggest levels of exposure that most employees may be exposed to for up to 10 hours per day, 40 hours per week, for a working lifetime, without experiencing adverse health effects. However, not all employees will be protected if their exposures are maintained below these levels. Some may have adverse health effects because of individual susceptibility, a pre-existing medical condition, or a hypersensitivity (allergy). In addition, some hazardous substances act in combination with other exposures, with the general environment, or with medications or personal habits of the employee to produce adverse health effects. Most OELs address airborne exposures, but some substances can be absorbed directly through the skin and mucous membranes.

Most OELs are expressed as a TWA exposure. A TWA refers to the average exposure during a normal 8- to 10-hour workday. Some chemical substances and physical agents have recommended short-term exposure limits (STELs) or ceiling values. Unless otherwise noted, the STEL is a 15-minute TWA exposure. It should not be exceeded at any time during a workday. The ceiling limit should not be exceeded at any time.

In the United States, OELs have been established by federal agencies, professional organizations, state and local governments, and other entities. Some OELs are legally enforceable limits; others are recommendations.

- The U.S. Department of Labor OSHA PELs (29 CFR 1910 [general industry]; 29 CFR 1926 [construction industry]; and 29 CFR 1917 [maritime industry]) are legal limits. These limits are enforceable in workplaces covered under the Occupational Safety and Health Act of 1970.

- NIOSH RELs are recommendations based on a critical review of the scientific and technical information and the adequacy of methods to identify and control the hazard. NIOSH RELs are published in the *NIOSH Pocket Guide to Chemical Hazards* [NIOSH 2010]. NIOSH also recommends risk management practices (e.g., engineering controls, safe work practices, employee education/training, personal protective equipment, and exposure and medical monitoring) to minimize the risk of exposure and adverse health effects.

- Other OELs commonly used and cited in the United States include the TLVs, which are recommended by ACGIH, a professional organization, and the WEELs, which are recommended by the American Industrial Hygiene Association, another professional organization. The TLVs and WEELs are developed by committee members of these associations from a review of the published, peer-reviewed literature. These OELs are not consensus standards. TLVs are considered voluntary exposure guidelines for use by industrial hygienists and others trained in this discipline "to assist in the control of health hazards" [ACGIH 2013]. WEELs have been established for some chemicals "when no other legal or authoritative limits exist" [AIHA 2012].

Outside the United States, OELs have been established by various agencies and organizations and include legal and recommended limits. The Institut für Arbeitsschutz der Deutschen Gesetzlichen Unfallversicherung (Institute for Occupational Safety and Health of the German Social Accident Insurance) maintains a database of international OELs from European Union member states, Canada (Québec), Japan, Switzerland, and the United States. The database, available at http://www.dguv.de/ifa/en/gestis/limit_values/index.jsp, contains international limits for more than 1,500 hazardous substances and is updated periodically.

OSHA requires an employer to furnish employees a place of employment free from recognized hazards that cause or are likely to cause death or serious physical harm [Occupational Safety and Health Act of 1970 (Public Law 91–596, sec. 5(a)(1))]. This is true in the absence of a specific OEL. It also is important to keep in mind that OELs may not reflect current health-based information.

When multiple OELs exist for a substance or agent, NIOSH investigators generally encourage employers to use the lowest OEL when making risk assessment and risk management decisions. NIOSH investigators also encourage use of the hierarchy of controls approach to eliminate or minimize workplace hazards. This includes, in order of preference, the use of (1) substitution or elimination of the hazardous agent, (2) engineering controls (e.g., local exhaust ventilation, process enclosure, dilution ventilation), (3) administrative controls (e.g., limiting time of exposure, employee training, work practice changes, medical surveillance), and (4) personal protective equipment (e.g., respiratory protection, gloves, eye protection, hearing protection). Control banding, a qualitative risk assessment and risk management tool, is a complementary approach to protecting employee health. Control banding focuses on how broad categories of risk should be managed. Information on control banding is available at http://www.cdc.gov/niosh/topics/ctrlbanding/. This approach can be applied in situations where OELs have not been established or can be used to supplement existing OELs.

Below we provide the OELs and surface contamination limits for the compounds we measured, as well as a discussion of the potential health effects from exposure to these compounds.

Formaldehyde

Under the OSHA general industry standard for airborne exposure to formaldehyde [29 CFR 1910.1048], the PEL is 0.75 ppm for an 8-hour TWA, the action level is 0.5 ppm for an 8-hour TWA, and the STEL is 2 ppm for a 15-minute TWA. The standard requires medical surveillance for employees exposed to formaldehyde at or above the action level or STEL.

The NIOSH REL for formaldehyde is 0.016 ppm for up to an 8-hour TWA. NIOSH also has a 15-minute ceiling limit of 0.1 ppm that is not to be exceeded during a work shift [NIOSH

2010]. NIOSH recognized formaldehyde as a potential occupational carcinogen in 1981 and, following the NIOSH carcinogen policy at the time, set the REL to the "lowest feasible concentration," which for formaldehyde was defined as the analytical limit of quantification of 0.016 ppm for up to 8 hours [NIOSH 1981]. Since then, experience has shown that this REL is actually not the "lowest feasible concentration" because formaldehyde in the ambient air can exceed 0.016 ppm, a fact later acknowledged by NIOSH [Lemen 1987]. Additionally, a revision of the NIOSH carcinogen policy [NIOSH 1995], combined with better exposure characterization and advances in risk assessment and management strategies, support the need for NIOSH to reassess the formaldehyde REL. This effort is in progress.

The ACGIH lists formaldehyde as a sensitizer with a ceiling limit of 0.3 ppm [ACGIH 2013]. An ACGIH ceiling limit is an exposure that should not be exceeded at any time during the work shift.

The International Agency for Research on Cancer classifies formaldehyde as a human carcinogen (group 1) on the basis of associations between formaldehyde exposure and nasopharyngeal cancer and leukemia [Baan et al. 2009]. NIOSH considers formaldehyde as a potential occupational carcinogen; ACGIH lists formaldehyde as a suspected human carcinogen; and the U.S. Department of Health and Human Services lists formaldehyde as reasonably anticipated to be a human carcinogen in its 11th report on carcinogens [NIOSH 1981; DHHS 2011; ACGIH 2013].

Volatile Organic Compounds

VOCs are a large class of low molecular weight chemicals that are organic (i.e., containing carbon) and have a sufficiently high vapor pressure to allow some of the compounds to exist in the gaseous state at room temperature. The health effects associated with VOCs depend on the toxicity of the specific VOC, the level of exposure, and the duration of the exposure [EPA 2012]. Symptoms from exposure to VOCs may include eye and respiratory tract irritation, headaches, dizziness, visual disorders, and memory impairment [NIOSH 2010]. The most common route of exposure to VOCs is through inhalation, but some solvents may contribute to systemic health effects through skin absorption [LaDou 1990; Klaassen 2008]. The rate of systemic elimination of solvents depends on how volatile and lipophilic the chemicals are. Some subpopulations may be more susceptible to health effects from solvents on the basis of age, sex, and genetics [Klaassen 2008]. VOCs are emitted in varying concentrations from numerous indoor sources including, but not limited to, carpeting, fabrics, adhesives, solvents, paints, cleaners, waxes, cigarettes, and combustion sources. Heating, burning, or chemical reactions may cause materials to emit VOCs. NIOSH and ACGIH have recommended occupational exposure limits for many VOCs [NIOSH 2010; ACGIH 2013]. OSHA also has standards or PELs for many VOCs [29 CFR 1910.1000].

Mold and Microbial Contamination

Exposure to microbes is not unique to the indoor environment. No environment, indoors or out, is completely free from microbes, even a surgical operating room. Remediation of microbial contamination may improve IEQ conditions even though a specific cause-effect relationship is not determined. NIOSH investigators routinely recommend the remediation of observed microbial contamination and the correction of situations that are favorable for microbial growth and bioaerosol dissemination.

The types and severity of symptoms related to exposure to mold in the indoor environment depend in part on the extent of the mold present, the extent of the individual's exposure, and the susceptibility of the individuals (for example, whether they have pre-existing allergies or asthma). In general, excessive exposure to fungi may produce health problems by several primary mechanisms, including allergy or hypersensitivity, infection, and toxic effects. Molds can trigger asthma symptoms (shortness of breath, wheezing, cough) in persons who are allergic to mold. Repeated or single exposure to mold or mold spores may cause previously nonsensitized individuals to become sensitized. Additionally, molds produce a variety of VOCs, the most common of which is ethanol, that have been postulated to cause upper airway irritation. However, potential irritant effects of VOCs from exposure to mold in the indoor environment are not well understood. Evidence also shows that exposure to fungal fragments that can contain allergens, toxins, and $(1\rightarrow3)$-β-D-glucan may occur [Górny et al. 2002; Brasel et al. 2005; Reponen et al. 2006].

In 2004, the Institute of Medicine (IOM) of the National Academies published a detailed review of previous scientific studies evaluating health effects of damp buildings [IOM 2004]. In 2009, the WHO published an updated review of this literature [WHO 2009]. These two documents highlight the respiratory health risks of exposure to damp indoor environments. The WHO report explains that: "the presence of many biological agents in the indoor environment is due to dampness and inadequate ventilation. Excess moisture on almost all indoor materials leads to growth of microbes, such as mold, fungi and bacteria, which subsequently emit spores, cells, fragments and volatile organic compounds into indoor air. Moreover, dampness initiates chemical or biological degradation of materials, which also pollutes indoor air." With respect to health effects from indoor dampness, the WHO report explains that there is sufficient epidemiologic evidence to conclude that occupants of damp buildings are at risk of developing upper and lower respiratory tract symptoms including cough, wheeze, respiratory infections, asthma, and exacerbation of asthma. The WHO report also stated limited evidence suggests an association between damp buildings and bronchitis and allergic rhinitis, and that there is clinical evidence that exposure to mold and other microbial agents in damp buildings increases the risk of hypersensitivity pneumonitis, chronic rhinosinusitis, and allergic fungal sinusitis. Additional evidence from a more recent epidemiologic review reported that bronchitis, shortness of breath and eczema should be added to the list of health outcomes with sufficient evidence of an association to dampness and dampness-related agents [Mendell et al. 2011].

People with weakened immune systems (immune-compromised or immune-suppressed individuals) may be more vulnerable to infections by molds. For example, *Aspergillus fumigatus* is a fungal species that has been found almost everywhere on every conceivable type of substrate. It has been known to infect the lungs of immune-compromised individuals who inhale the airborne spores [Wald and Stave 1994; Brandt et al. 2006]. Healthy individuals are usually not vulnerable to infections from airborne mold exposure.

No standards specific to the nonindustrial indoor environment exist. Measurement of indoor environmental contaminants has seldom proved helpful in determining the cause of symptoms except where there are unusual sources or a proven relationship between specific exposures and disease. With few exceptions, concentrations of frequently measured chemical substances in the indoor work environment fall well below the recommended OELs published by NIOSH [NIOSH 2010], ACGIH [ACGIH 2013], and the American Industrial Hygiene Association [AIHA 2012], and the mandatory PELs set by OSHA [29 CFR 1910 (general industry)]. ANSI/ASHRAE has published recommended building thermal comfort and ventilation guidelines [ANSI/ASHRAE/ASHE 2008; ANSI/ASHRAE 2010a,b]. ACGIH and American Industrial Hygiene Association have also developed a manual of guidelines for approaching investigations of building-related symptoms that might be caused by airborne living organisms or their effluents [ACGIH 1999; AIHA 2008]. Other resources that provide guidance for establishing acceptable IEQ are available through U.S. EPA at http://www.epa.gov/iaq/, especially the joint U.S. EPA/NIOSH document, Building Air Quality, A Guide for Building Owners and Facility Managers at http://www.epa.gov/iaq/largebldgs/baqtoc.html.

Temperature and Relative Humidity

Temperature and relative humidity measurements are often collected as part of an IEQ evaluation because these parameters affect the perception of comfort in an indoor environment. The perception of thermal comfort is related to one's metabolic heat production, the transfer of heat to the environment, physiological adjustments, and body temperature [NIOSH 1986]. Heat transfer from the body to the environment is influenced by factors such as temperature, humidity, air movement, personal activities, and clothing. The ANSI/ASHRAE Standard 55-2010, *Thermal Environmental Conditions for Human Occupancy*, specifies conditions in which 80% or more of the occupants would be expected to find the environment thermally acceptable [ANSI/ASHRAE 2010a]. Assuming slow air movement and 50% relative humidity, the operative temperatures recommended by ANSI/ASHRAE range from 68.5°F–76°F in the winter, and from 75°F–80.5°F in the summer. The difference between the two is largely due to seasonal clothing selection. ANSI/ASHRAE also recommends that relative humidity be maintained at or below 65% [ANSI/ASHRAE 2010a]. Excessive humidity can promote the excessive growth of microorganisms and dust mites. The ASHRAE/ASHE Standard 170-2008, *Ventilation in Health Care Facilities*, specifies ventilation design parameters that provide control of environmental comfort, asepsis, and odor for spaces commonly found in health care facilities. For general laboratories and histology laboratories, ventilation systems should be capable of maintaining a range of 70°F–75°F during normal operations. For autopsy rooms, the recommended temperature range is 68°F–75°F. No relative humidity range recommendations are provided for these areas [ANSI/ASHRAE/ASHE 2008].

References

ACGIH [1999]. Bioaerosols: assessment and control. Cincinnati, OH: American Conference of Governmental Industrial Hygienists.

ACGIH [2013]. 2013 TLVs® and BEIs®: threshold limit values for chemical substances and physical agents and biological exposure indices. Cincinnati, OH: American Conference of Governmental Industrial Hygienists.

AIHA [2008]. Recognition, evaluation, and control of indoor mold. Prezant B, Weekes DM, Miller JD, eds. Fairfax, VA: American Industrial Hygiene Association.

AIHA [2012]. AIHA 2012 Emergency response planning guidelines (ERPG) & workplace environmental exposure levels (WEEL) handbook. Fairfax, VA: American Industrial Hygiene Association.

ANSI/ASHRAE [2010a]. Thermal environmental conditions for human occupancy. American National Standards Institute/ASHRAE standard 55-2010. Atlanta, GA: American Society for Heating, Refrigerating, and Air-Conditioning Engineers, Inc.

ANSI/ASHRAE [2010b]. Ventilation for acceptable indoor air quality. American National Standards Institute/ASHRAE standard 62.1-2010. Atlanta, GA: American Society of Heating, Refrigerating, and Air-Conditioning Engineers, Inc.

ANSI/ASHRAE/ASHE [2008]. Ventilation of health care facilities. American National Standards Institute/ASHRAE/American Society of Healthcare Engineering standard 170-2008. Atlanta, GA: American Society of Heating, Refrigerating, and Air-Conditioning Engineers, Inc.

ASHRAE [2011]. 2011 ASHRAE handbook: HVAC applications. Health-care facilities. Atlanta, GA: American Society for Heating, Refrigerating, and Air-Conditioning Engineers, Inc.

Baan R, Grosse Y, Straif K, Secretan B, El Ghissassi F, Bouvard V, Benbrahim-Tallaa L, Guha N, Freeman C, Galichet L, Cogliano V, on the behalf of the WHO International Agency for Research on Cancer Monograph Working Group [2009]. A review of human carcinogens-Part F: chemical agents and related occupations. Lancet Oncol 10(12):1143–1144.

Brandt M, Brown C, Burkhart J, Burton N, Cox-Ganser J, Damon S, Falk H, Fridkin S, Garbe P, McGeehin M, Morgan J, Page E, Rao C, Redd S, Sinks T, Trout D, Wallingford K, Warnock D, Weissman D [2006]. Mold prevention strategies and possible health effects in the aftermath of hurricanes and major floods. MMWR 55(RR-8):1–27.

Brasel TL, Martin JM, Carriker CG, Wilson SC, Straus DC [2005]. Detection of airborne Stachybotrys chartarum macrocyclic trichothecene mycotoxins in the indoor environment. Appl Environ Microbiol 71(11):7376–7388.

CDC [2012]. Guidelines for safe work practices in human and animal medical diagnostic laboratories. MMWR *61*(1):38–46.

CFR. Code of Federal Regulations. Washington, DC: U.S. Government Printing Office, Office of the Federal Register.

DHHS [2011]. Addendum to the 12th report on carcinogens. U.S. Department of Health and Human Services, National Toxicology Program. [http://ntp.niehs.nih.gov/ntp/roc/twelfth/Addendum.pdf]. Date accessed: June 2013.

EPA [2001]. Mold remediation in schools and commercial buildings. Washington, DC: United States Environmental Protection Agency, Office of Air and Radiation, Indoor Environments Division. EPA Publication No. 402–K–01–001.

EPA [2012]. An introduction to indoor air quality: organic gases (volatile organic compounds – VOCs). [http://www.epa.gov/iaq/voc.html]. Date accessed: June 2013.

Facility Guidelines Institute [2010]. Guidelines for design and construction of health care facilities, 2010 edition. Chicago, IL: American Society of Healthcare Engineering of the American Hospital Association.

Górny RL, Reponen T, Willeke K, Schmechel D, Robine E, Boissier M, Grinshpun SA [2002]. Fungal fragments as indoor air biocontaminants. Appl Environ Microbiol *68*(7):3522–3531.

Green F, Yoshida K [1990]. Characteristics of aerosols generated during autopsy procedures and their potential role as carriers of infectious agents. Occup Environ Hyg *5*(12):853–858.

IOM [2004]. Damp indoor spaces and health. Washington, DC: Institute of Medicine, National Academy Press.

Klaassen CD, ed. [2008]. Casarett and Doull's toxicology: the basic science of poisons. 7th ed. New York: McGraw-Hill Companies, Inc. pp. 931–997.

LaDou J [1990]. Occupational medicine. Norwalk, CT: Appleton & Lange, pp. 297–326.

Lemen RA [1987]. Official letter from R.A. Lemen, Director, Division of Standards Development and Technology Transfer, National Institute for Occupational Safety and Health, U.S. Department of Health and Human Services, Cincinnati, OH to Tom Hall, Docket Office, Department of Labor, Washington, DC, February 9.

Mendell MJ, Mirer AG, Cheung K, Tong M, Douwes J [2011]. Respiratory and allergic health effects of dampness, mold and dampness-related agents: a review of the epidemiologic evidence. Environ Health Perspect *119*(6):748–756.

Newman LS, Rose CS, Bresnitz EA, Rossman MD, Barnard J, Frederick M, Terrin ML, Weinberger SE, Moller DR, McLennan G, Hunninghake G, DePalo L, Baughman RP, Iannuzzi MC, Judson MA, Knatterud GL, Thompson BW, Teirstein AS, Yeager H Jr, Johns CJ, Rabin DL, Rybicki BA, Cherniack R, ACCESS Research Group [2004]. A case control etiologic study of sarcoidosis: environmental and occupational risk factors. Am J Respir Crit Care Med *170*(12):1324–1330.

Newman KL, Newman LS [2012]. Occupational causes of sarcoidosis. Opin Allergy Clin Immunol *12*(2):145–150.

NIOSH [1981]. Current intelligence bulletin 34 – formaldehyde: evidence of carcinogenicity. Cincinnati, OH: U.S. Department of Health and Human Services, Centers for Disease Control, National Institute for Occupational Safety and Health. DHHS (NIOSH) Publication No. DHHS (NIOSH) 81-111 (1981, updated 1997).

NIOSH [1986]. Criteria for a recommended standard: occupational exposure to hot environments, revised criteria. Cincinnati, OH: U.S. Department of Health and Human Services, Centers for Disease Control, National Institute for Occupational Safety and Health, DHHS (NIOSH) Publication No. 86-13.

NIOSH [1995]. NIOSH recommended exposure limit policy. September 1995. In: NIOSH policy statements. Cincinnati, OH: U.S. Department of Health and Human Services, Centers for Disease Control and Prevention, National Institute for Occupational Safety and Health.

NIOSH [1997a]. NIOSH Alert: Preventing allergic reactions to natural rubber latex in the workplace. Cincinnati, OH: U.S. Department of Health and Human Services, Centers for Disease Control and Prevention, National Institute for Occupational Safety and Health, DHHS (NIOSH) Report No. 97-135.

NIOSH [1997b]. Hazard evaluation and technical assistance report: Los Angeles County Department of Coroner – Los Angeles, California. By Martinez K and Tubbs R. Cincinnati, OH: U.S. Department of Health and Human Services, Centers for Disease Control and Prevention, National Institute for Occupational Safety and Health, NIOSH HETA No. 1996-0019-2666.

NIOSH [2010]. NIOSH pocket guide to chemical hazards. Cincinnati, OH: U.S. Department of Health and Human Services, Centers for Disease Control and Prevention, National Institute for Occupational Safety and Health, DHHS (NIOSH) Publication No. 2010-168c. [http://www.cdc.gov/niosh/npg/]. Date accessed: June 2013.

NIOSH [2012]. NIOSH alert: preventing occupational respiratory disease from exposures caused by dampness in office buildings, schools, and other nonindustrial buildings. By Martin M, Cox-Ganser J, Kreiss K, Kanwal R, and Sahakian N. Cincinnati, OH: U.S. Department of Health and Human Services, Centers for Disease Control and Prevention,

National Institute for Occupational Safety and Health, DHHS (NIOSH) Publication No. 2013-102.

Nolte K, Taylor D, Richmond J [2002]. Biosafety consideration for autopsy. Am J Forensic Med Pathol 23(2):107–122.

NRC [1981]. Formaldehyde and other aldehydes. Washington, DC: National Research Council (National Academy Press).

Redd SC [2002]. State of the science on molds and human health. Statement for the Record Before the Subcommittee on Oversight and Investigations and Housing and Community Opportunity, Committee on Financial Services, United States House of Representatives. Atlanta, GA: U.S. Department of Health and Human Services, Centers for Disease Control and Prevention.

Reponen T, Seo S-C, Iossifova Y, Adhikari A, Grinshpun SA [2006]. New field-compatible method for collection and analysis of β-glucan in fungal fragments. Abstracts of the International Aerosol Conference, St. Paul, Minnesota, p. 955.

Rosenstock L [1996]. NIOSH Testimony to the U.S. Department of Labor on indoor air quality. Appl Occup Environ Hyg 11(12):1365–1370.

Rossman MD, Thompson B, Frederick M, Iannuzzi MC, Rybicki BA, Pander JP, Newman LS, Rose C, Magira E, Monos D, ACCESS Group [2008]. HLA and environmental interactions in sarcoidosis. Sarcoidosis Vasc Diffuse Lung Dis 25(2):125–132.

Wald P, Stave G [1994]. Fungi. In: Physical and biological hazards of the workplace. New York: Van Nostrand Reinhold, p. 394.

WHO [2009]. WHO guidelines for indoor air quality: dampness and mould. Geneva, Switzerland: World Health Organization. [http://www.euro.who.int/document/e92645.pdf]. Date accessed: June 2013.

Keywords: NAICS 923120 (Administration of Public Health Programs), coroner, medical examiner, autopsies, histology, formaldehyde, IEQ, mold, chemical, ventilation, fiberglass, latex gloves

The Health Hazard Evaluation Program investigates possible health hazards in the workplace under the authority of Section 20(a)(6) of the Occupational Safety and Health Act of 1970, 29 U.S.C. 669(a)(6). The Health Hazard Evaluation Program also provides, upon request, technical assistance to federal, state, and local agencies to control occupational health hazards and to prevent occupational illness and disease. Regulations guiding the Program can be found in Title 42, Code of Federal Regulations, Part 85; Requests for Health Hazard Evaluations (42 CFR 85).

Acknowledgments

Analytical Support: Jennifer Roberts, Bureau Veritas North America, and Microbiology Specialists Incorporated
Desktop Publishers: Mary Winfree
Editor: Ellen Galloway
Health Communicator: Stefanie Brown
Industrial Hygiene Field Assistance: Chad Dowell
Logistics: Donnie Booher and Karl Feldmann

Availability of Report

Copies of this report have been sent to the employer, employees, and union at the facility. The state and local health department and the Occupational Safety and Health Administration Regional Office have also received a copy. This report is not copyrighted and may be freely reproduced.

This report is available at http://www.cdc.gov/niosh/hhe/reports/pdfs/2012-0135-3184.pdf.